12 MINUTES TO:

HEALTHY BACKS

JOANIE GREGGAINS

Contoure
IN TUNE WITH YOUR BODY

Use your phone or tablet to scan the QR code and click on the URL to listen to the Word-for-Word Audio Read-Along.

CONGRATULATIONS, you have chosen a wonderful exercise program to help you have a healthier, happier back.

YOU are only 12 MINUTES away from having a BETTER BACK.

Your back works 24 hours a day. It even works when you're asleep. When you're awake it carries all of the responsibility for your upright position. No wonder it's sore.

These exercises will help to stretch, strengthen, and straighten your backs. You might even stand a little taller, and you should notice an improvement in your posture. No more slumping over.

So, let's get started. I know that you can't wait for your back to feel better.

Remember, to use slow easy movements when you do these exercises. Be careful of your back by doing all of the exercises smoothly. I have also included some exercises that strengthen your abdominal muscles, because they can help the back.

Make sure that you have enough room to exercise. Wear loose clothing, and exercise on a mat or a soft carpet.

If you experience any unusual pain or if you've had any back problems consult your physician. Always consult your physician before starting any exercise program.

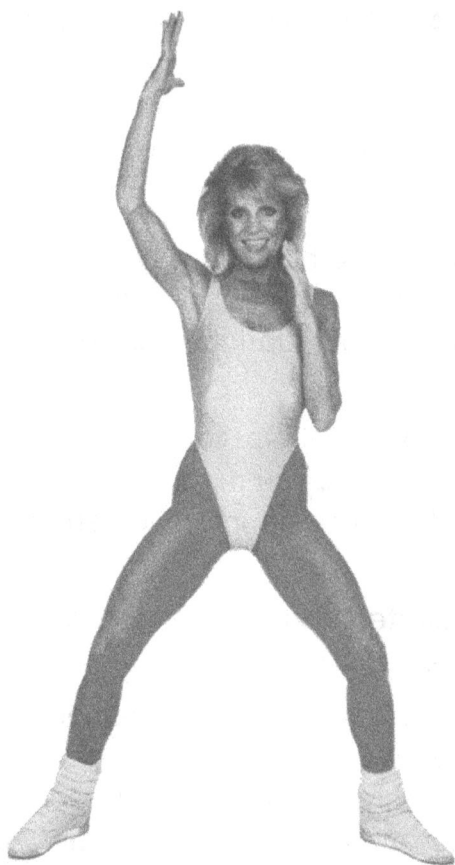

1. HEAVEN STRETCH—Stand with your legs slightly bent and the palms of your hands turned in towards each other. Alternate raising the left hand and the right. Pull through the spine, keeping your abdominal muscles tight. The motion should be like climbing a rope. Do this for approximately 1 minute.

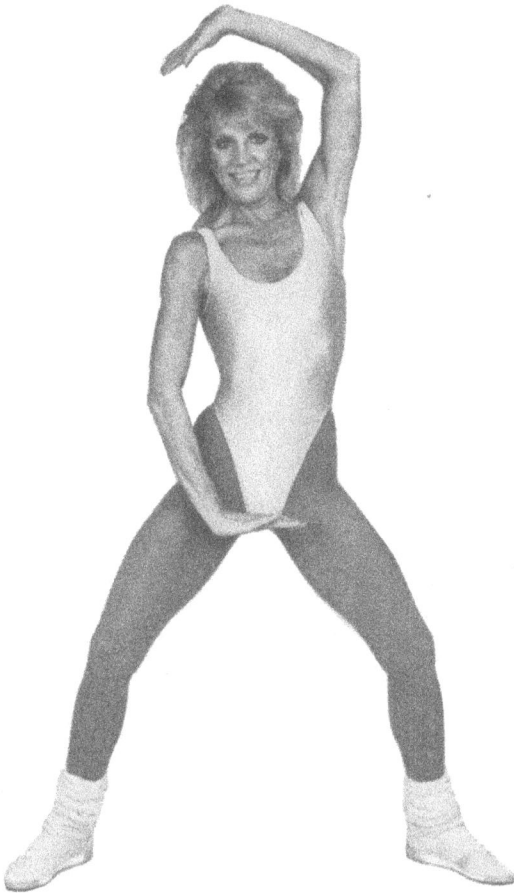

2. HEAVEN PRESS—The position is the same as in the **HEAVEN STRETCH**, but this time turn the palms upward as you press towards the ceiling. Do this for approximately 30 seconds.

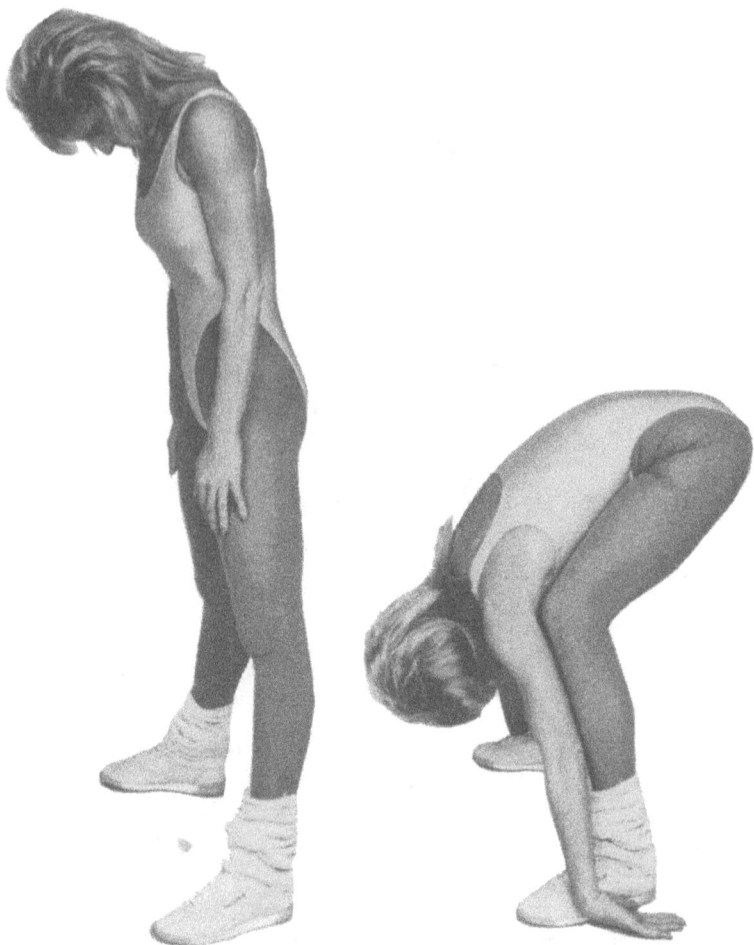

3. SPINAL ROLL—Now bring your chin to your chest, and slowly lower your body down to your knees. Then roll slowly upward vertebra by vertebra. Do this for approximately 1 minute.

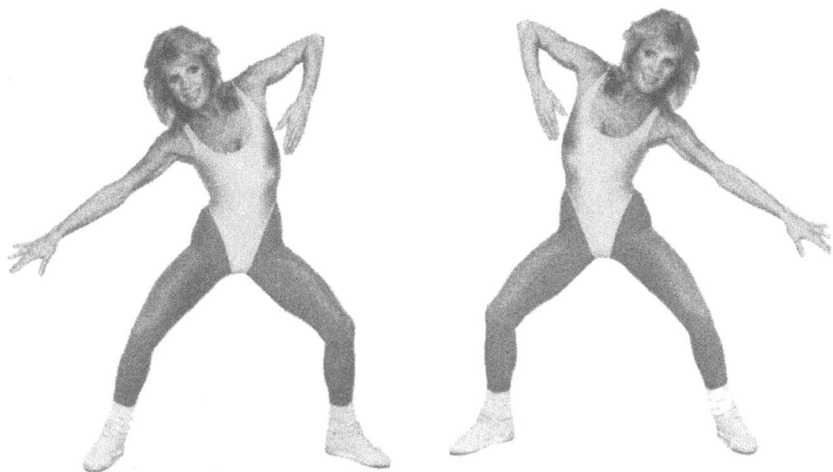

4. TORSO BEND—Place the feet wider than shoulder width apart, and slightly bend the knees. The left arm is up and bent towards the body, and the right arm is reaching outward. Alternate right and left, while tightening your abdominal muscles. Stretch side to side for approximately 1 minute.

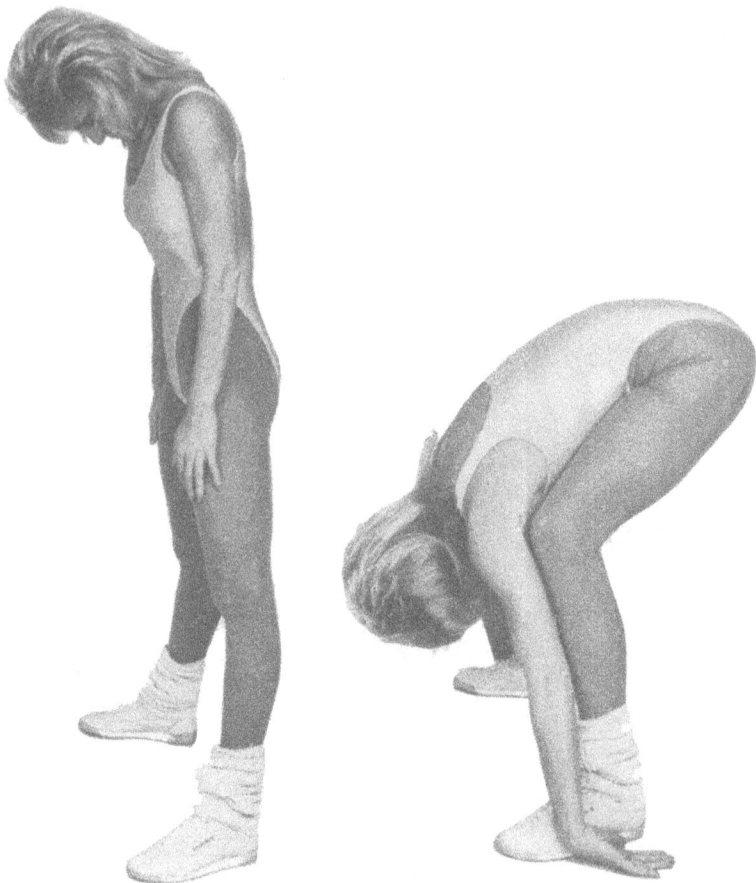

5. SPINAL ROLL—Now bring your chin to your chest, and slowly lower your body down to your knees. Then roll slowly upward vertebra by vertebra. Do this for approximately 1 minute.

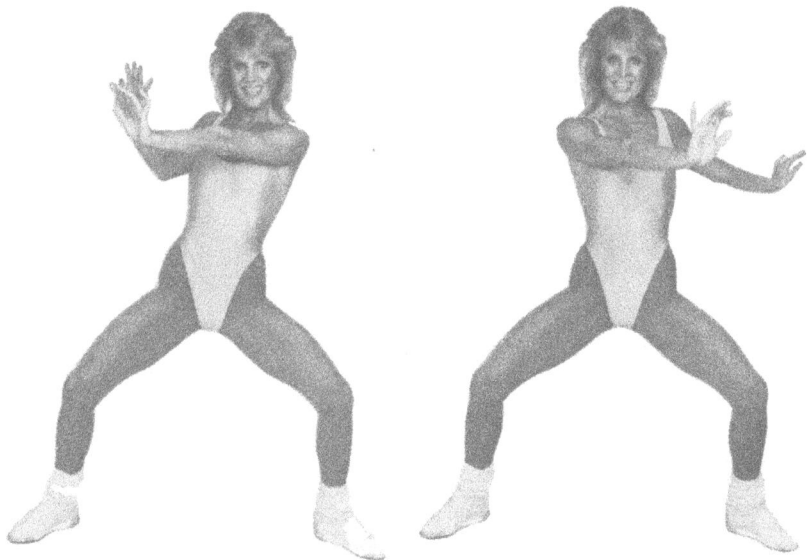

6. WAIST TWIST—Stand with your legs apart in a slight squat position. Keep your spine straight and twist from side to side by shifting your arms from one side to the other. Do this for approximately 1 minute.

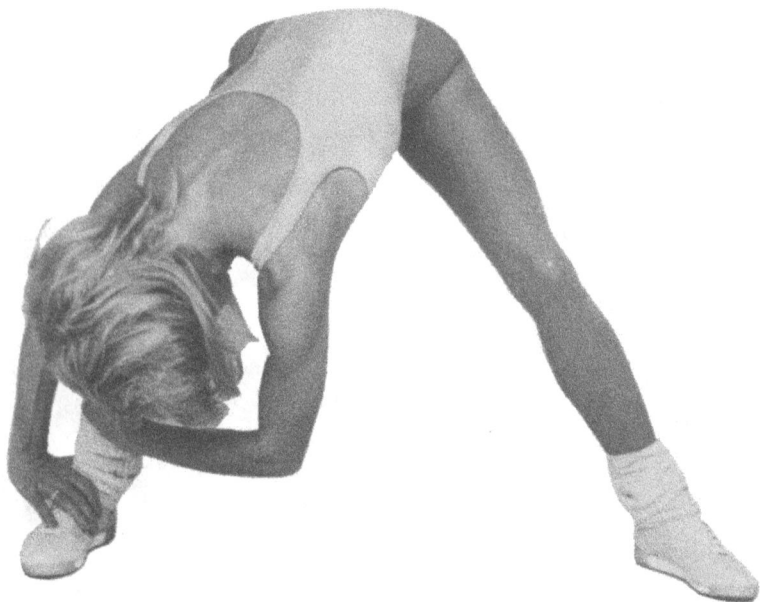

7. LOWER LEG HOLD—Now bend over to the floor and bend the right knee as you hold onto the right ankle. Try to keep the left leg straight. Pulse for approximately 30 seconds. Then switch sides and pulse holding onto the left ankle for approximately 30 seconds. (Now release and go down to the floor. Lie comfortably on your back.)

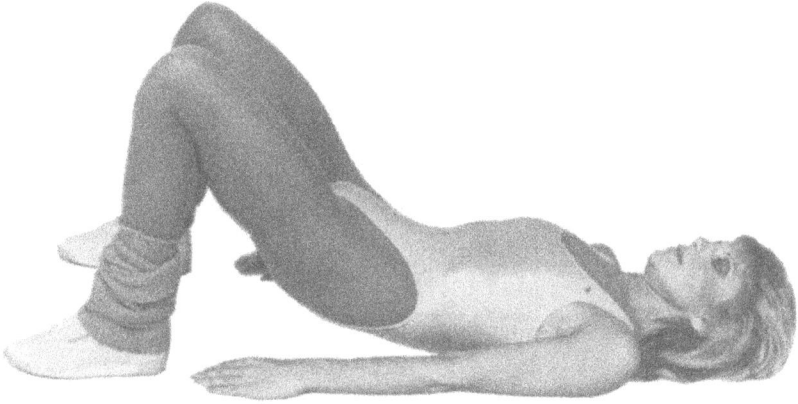

8. PELVIC TILT—Lie with your back on the floor. Your knees are bent, and your feet are on the floor. Press off the heels and lift your pelvic area towards the ceiling. Tighten the gluteus muscles as you press towards the ceiling. Press upward for approximately 45 seconds.

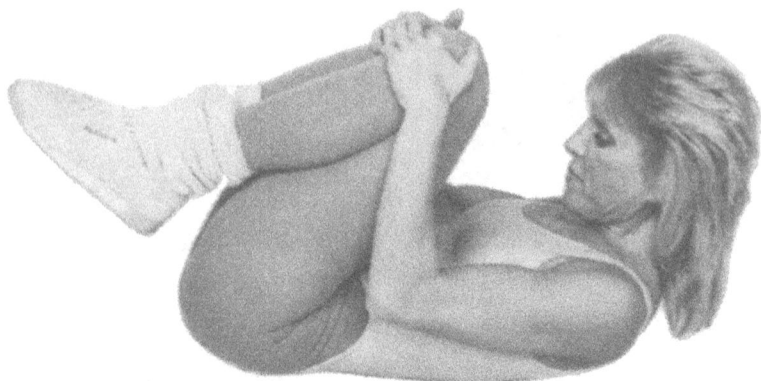

9. HUG KNEES—Bring your knees to your chest, and hug your knees as you roll from side to side. This massages the back, and will make it feel wonderful. Do this for approximately 25 seconds.

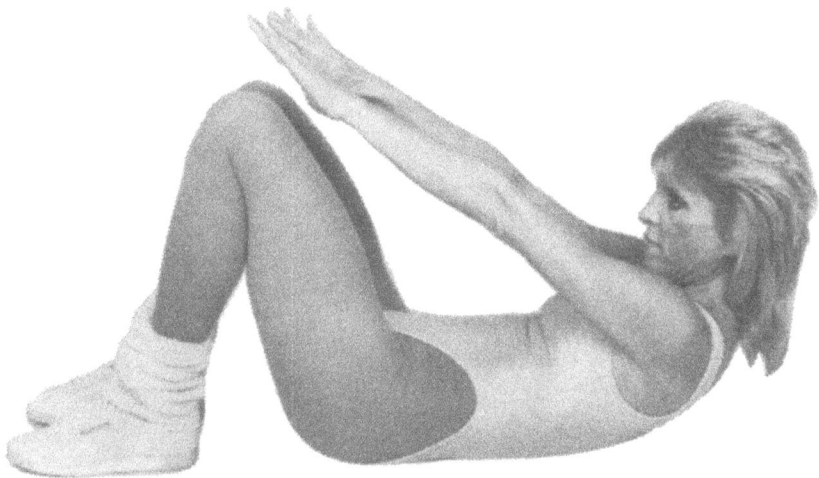

10. AB CURL—Now lie flat on your back with your knees bent and your feet on the floor. Keep your arms straight and pulse upward towards the knees. Just do little pulses. Try to exhale on the upward pulse and inhale on the downward pulse. Remember strong abdominal muscles help your back. Do this for approximately 45 seconds.

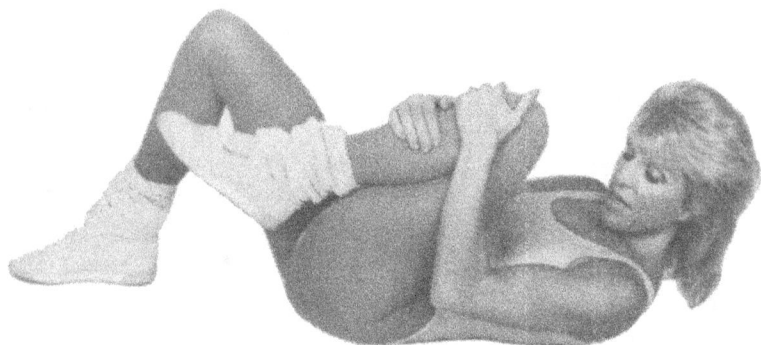

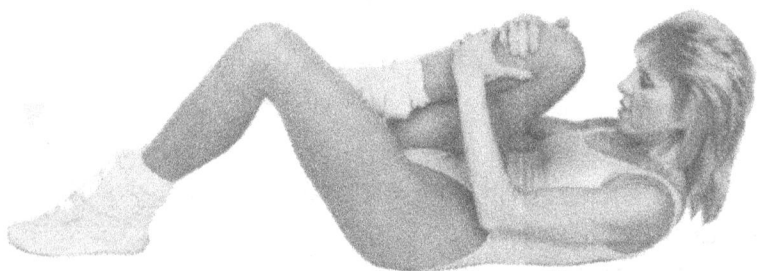

11. KNEE PRESS—Bring your right knee in towards your head, and hug it as you breathe deeply. Try to keep your back flat. Do this for approximately 30 seconds on the right side. Now switch to the left side and hug the left knee for approximately 30 seconds.

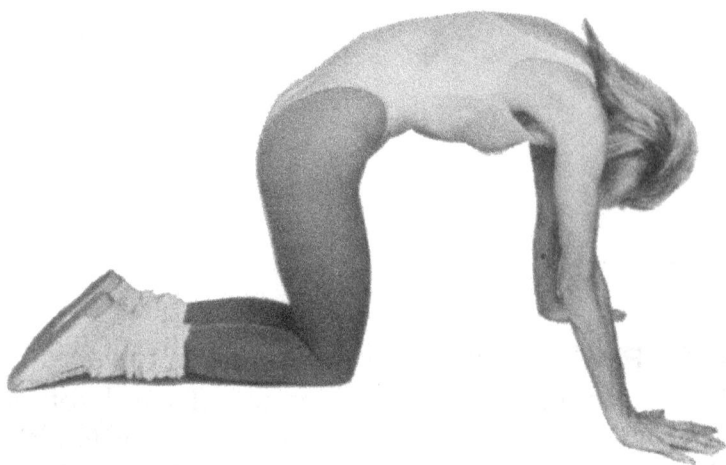

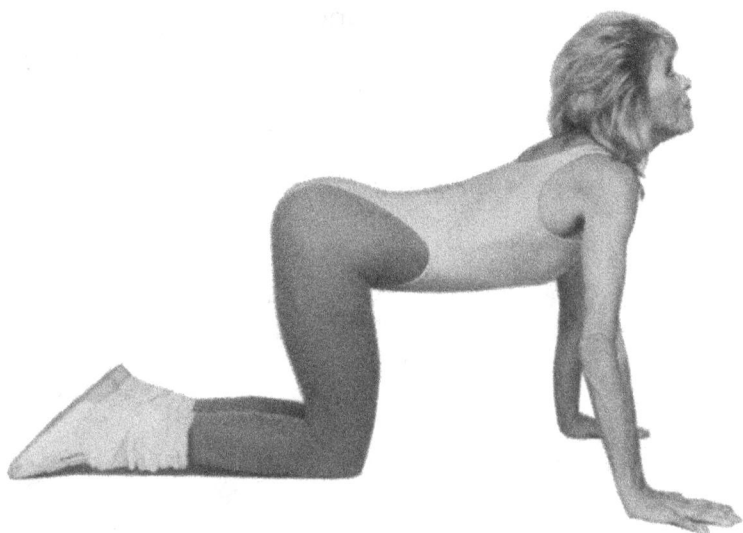

12. CAT STRETCH-—Now roll over and get onto your hands and knees. Pull inward with the abdominal muscles and curve the back upward. Relax the back, and then press downward with the back muscles so that you are making the back into a "U" shape. Alternate arching and making a "U" of the back. Do this for approximately 1 minute.

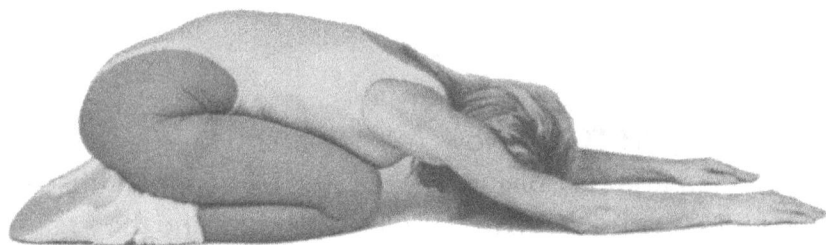

13. ENERGY STRETCH—Now rest backward so that you're seated on your heels. Stretch your arms straight out in front of you. Roll your head downward. Do this for approximately 30 seconds.

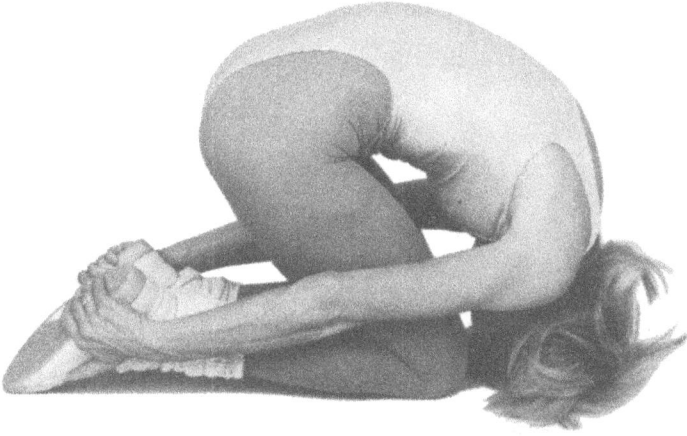

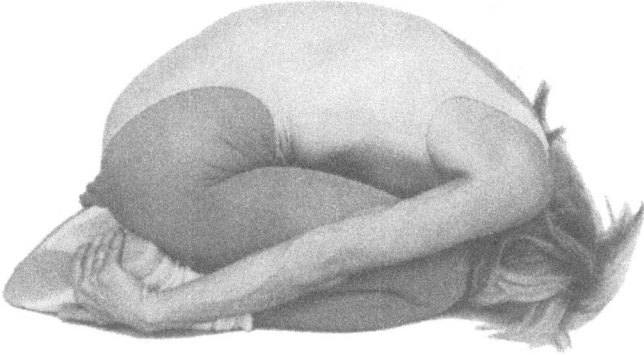

14. BABY BACK STRETCH—While seated on your heels hold onto the soles of your feet. Bring your head into your knees and lift your gluteals from your heels. Do this for approximately 30 seconds.

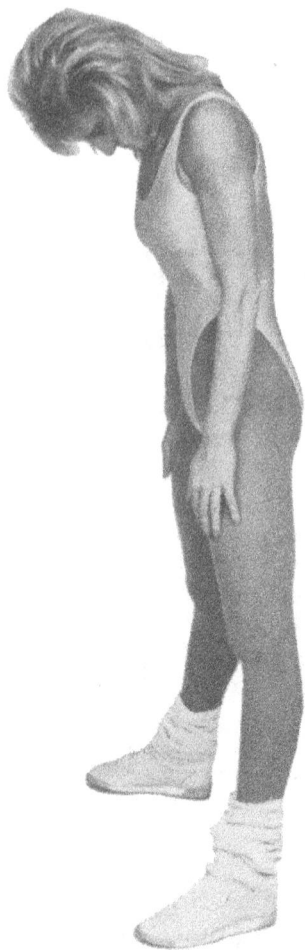
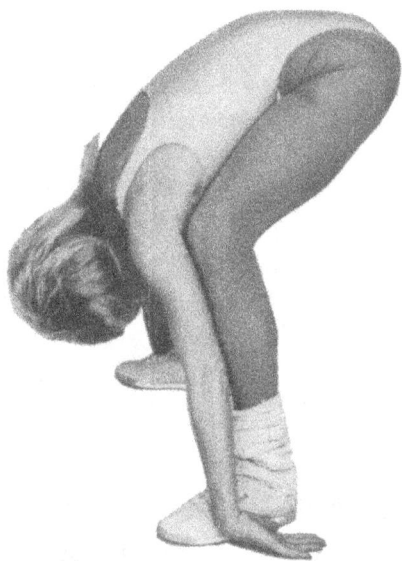

15. SPINAL ROLL—Now bring your chin to your chest, and slowly lower your body down to your knees. Then roll slowly upward vertebra by vertebra. Do this for approximately 1 minute.

Now doesn't your back feel wonderful? I know it does, because you've stretched and strengthened all of those sore muscles. Remember to do this 12 MINUTE WORK OUT 3 to 5 times a week, and when your back gets stronger you might want to repeat the tape twice in a row.

Look for my other 12 MINUTE WORK OUTS to strengthen, tone, and firm other specific body parts.

For a complete work out get my new video tape "Vital, Vigorous and Visual" It's available wherever video tapes are sold. Ask for it by name. Or you may want to consider getting one of my 3 best selling albums. Each one earned a gold record. They are all complete work outs from head to toe. They 're Fantastic! Look and ask for them wherever records or tapes are sold.

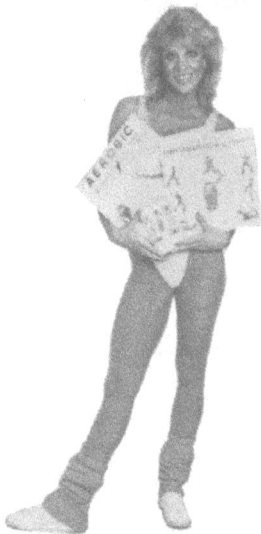

Also Available in the The Contoure Fitness Instructional books and recordings/audiobooks series

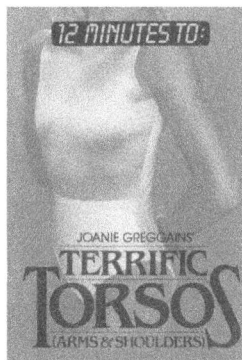

Terrific Torsos

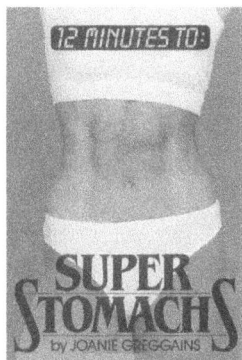

Super Stomachs

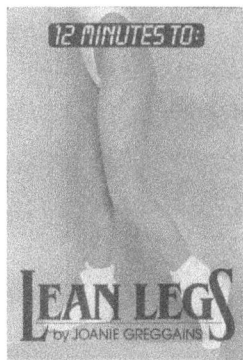

Lean Legs

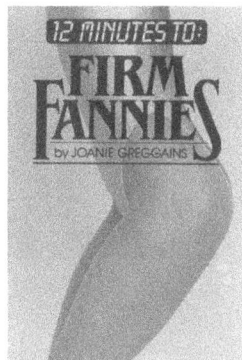

Firm Fannies

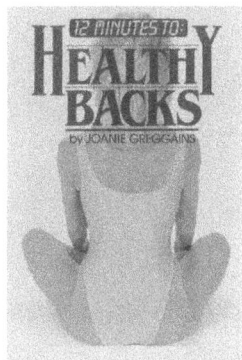

Healthy Backs

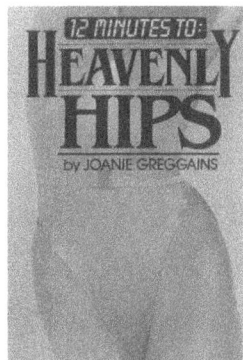

Heavenly Hips

Also Available in the The Contoure Fitness Instructional books and recordings/audiobooks series

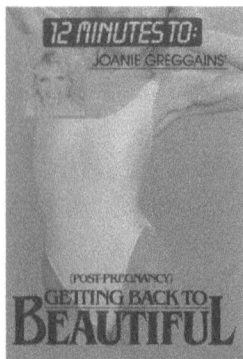

Getting Back To Beautiful

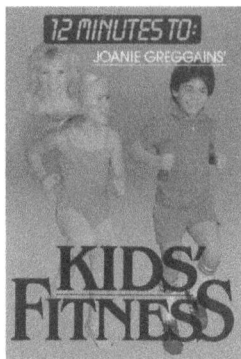

Kids' Fitness

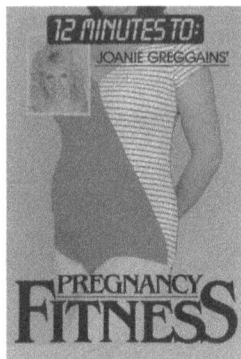

Pregnancy Fitness

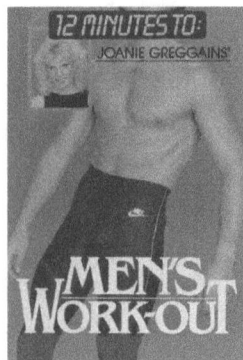

Men's Workout

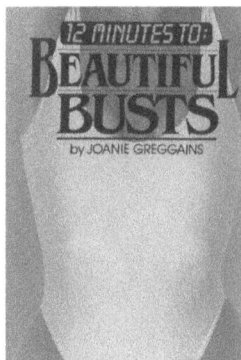

Beautiful Busts

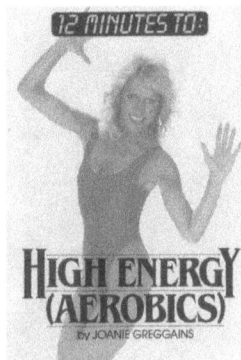

High Energy Aerobics

www.ingramcontent.com/pod-product-compliance
Lightning Source LLC
Chambersburg PA
CBHW072158020426
42334CB00018B/2060